End

Of

Alzheimer

Cookbook:

Recipes to help in Reversing Cognitive Impairment and Alzheimer's Disease.

By

Dave Miller

Disclaimer:

The information provided in this book is designed to provide helpful information on the subjects discussed. The publisher and author are not responsible for any specific health or allergy needs that may require medical supervision and are not liable for any damages or negative consequences from any treatment, action, application or preparation, to any person reading or following the information in this book.

Table of Contents

INTRODUCTIONS:

It is Time to Put an End to Alzheimer's Disease

Alzheimer's disease is the major cause of age-related cognitive decline, with over five (5) million Americans and thirty (30) million people globally suffering from the disorder. I pulled these numbers from the study recently conducted and they are probably even higher now.

Dementia has been recorded as the third leading cause of death in the United States behind cardiovascular disease and cancer, and by 2050, it's estimated that thirteen (13) million Americans and one hundred and sixty (160) million people globally will be affected by the disease (82).

However, we clearly need an effective prevention and treatment strategy, and conventional medicine is failing to deliver.

It is obvious that Bredesen's ideas have already begun to send shock waves throughout the medical community or at least that alert subset who make the effort both to continue their clinical education and to venture outside of classical medical school training. There are those who dismiss his ideas, but they make so much sense to me (as well as to a lot of folks much smarter than I) and offer both affordable and immediately applicable therapeutic interventions unlike any other research or reasoning in this field during my lifetime.

This cookbook is packed with mind blowing recipes to help in reversing cognitive impairment and Alzheimer's disease. This book can be a bit of slog at times even compared to similar titles that have come out this year like The Plant Paradox by Steven Gundry, undoctored by William Davis, and Head Strong by Dave Asprey but most importantly this only reflects the extent of Dr. Bredesen's research and intellect.

Undoubtedly, this book is worth the effort for anyone touched by someone experiencing or at risk for (pretty much everyone) cognitive decline. The recipes in this book apply Bredesen's approach broadly to any and all dementias be they officially diagnosed as Alzheimer's or not.

If you want to prevent and reverse cognitive decline, the first thing you should do is avoid processed food that contains refined carbohydrates (like flour and sugar) because they increase inflammation and cause blood sugar fluctuations.

Finally, this cookbook contains a bunch of healthy brain-boosting foods that you can eat on a regular basis.

Recipes to help in Reversing Cognitive Impairment and Alzheimer's Disease.

Blueberry Avocado Smoothie

Ingredients:

Avocado

Chia seeds

Ice

Blueberries

Banana

Pomegranate juice

Directions:

1. First, you place all ingredients in a blender.
2. Then you blend until smooth.

California Barley Bowl

Ingredients:

1 cup of bean sprouts

¼ cup of sliced almonds (toasted)

1 small ripe avocado (peeled, pitted, and diced or sliced)

Ground pepper

½ cup of cooked barley

1/3 cup of Cotija cheese (or better still queso fresco)

¼ teaspoon of kosher salt

Flaky salt

Ingredients for Lemony Yogurt Sauce:

1 teaspoon of grated lemon zest

Pinch of kosher salt

½ cup of plain yogurt

1 teaspoon of lemon juice

1 tablespoon of chopped chives

Directions:

1. First, you stir barley, cheese, sprouts, almonds and kosher salt together.
2. After which you whisk all yogurt sauce ingredients in a small both and refrigerate up to 3 days.
3. After that, you scoop barley mixture into two bowls, top with avocado and yogurt sauce.
4. Then you add salt and pepper to taste, serve.

Quinoa Avocado Sushi

Ingredients:

2 cups of water

1 teaspoon of maple syrup

1 small cucumber

4 sheets of nori sushi wrap

1 cup of quinoa

3 tablespoons of brown rice vinegar

Pinch of salt

Handful of spinach

One avocado

Directions:

1. First, you place quinoa and water in a saucepan.
2. After which you boil and then reduce heat to simmer until quinoa is cooked.
3. After that, you cut avocado and cucumber into thin strips.
4. Then you mix together maple syrup, vinegar, and salt in a small bowl.
5. At this point, you gradually pour vinegar mixture over quinoa, mixing as you pour.
6. This when you spread quinoa on each sushi wrap, leaving 2 inches at the end of each wrap.
7. Furthermore, you place spinach on quinoa and top with cucumber and avocado.
8. Finally, you roll up tightly and cut into rolls.

Asparagus, Snap Pea, and Avocado Pasta

Ingredients:

1 pound of asparagus (ends trimmed and cut into 2-inch lengths)

1 pound of bow-tie pasta (farfalle)

2 cloves garlic (minced)

½ cup of shredded Parmesan (or preferably pecorino cheese, plus more for serving, if desired)

Coarse salt and ground pepper

1 pound of sugar snap peas (strings removed)

4 tablespoons of butter

1 ripe avocado (halved, pitted, peeled, and cut into 1/2-inch chunks)

½ cup of chopped fresh mint (parsley, or preferably basil)

Directions:

1. First, you cook asparagus in boiling water for about two minutes.
2. After which you add snap peas, cook for 30 seconds then transfer asparagus and snap peas to a bowl.
3. After that, you return water to boil and add pasta.
4. Then you cook until al dente.
5. At this point, you drain and reserve 1 cup pasta water, set pasta aside.
6. Furthermore, melt 2 tablespoons butter over medium heat in a pasta pot.
7. After that, you add asparagus, snap peas and garlic.
8. After which you cook until vegetables are crisp.
9. This is when you add remaining butter, herbs, cooked pasta, avocado, cheese and reserved pasta water.
10. Finally, you toss to combine and season with salt, pepper, and cheese.

Caprese Stuffed Avocado

Ingredients:

8 oz. or ½ pound of mozzarella pearls or preferably ciliegine

4 avocados

Salt and pepper (to taste)

1 pint of cherry or preferably grape tomatoes (cut in halves)

½ cup of basil garlic oil sauce (adjust to taste)

Lettuce or salad greens to serve with the avocados (it is optional)

4 – 6 tablespoons of balsamic vinegar reduction sauce to drizzle (adjust to taste)

Directions:

Direction for the tomato caprese filling:

1. First, you place tomatoes, mozzarella pearls in a bowl with basil oil and mix well.
2. Remember it can be used immediately or refrigerated until ready to assemble.

Directions for the caprese stuffed avocados:

1. First, you cut the avocados in half lengthwise.
2. After which you remove pits and peel.
3. After that, you spoon filling into the avocado halves.
4. Then you drizzle with balsamic vinegar reduction and serve immediately.

Tuna Avocado Lettuce Wraps

Ingredients:

½ very ripe avocado

¼ cup of green olives

2 large leaves of green leaf lettuce

1 can of tuna

2 tablespoons of mayo

2 tablespoons of diced green chiles

1 scallion

Directions:

1. First, you cut olives in half and diced scallion.
2. After which you mash avocado until creamy, then mix with mayo.
3. After that, you add tuna, olives, scallion, and chives to the avocado mayo mixture.
4. Then you place one scoop of tuna salad on a lettuce leaf and enjoy!

Avocado and White Bean Salad with Vinaigrette

Ingredients:

Ingredients for the Salad

1 avocado (chopped)

¼ sweet onion chopped (optional)

1 can white beans

1 Roma tomato (chopped)

Ingredients for Vinaigrette:

¼ cup of lemon juice

Garlic powder (to taste)

1 teaspoon of mustard

1 ½ tablespoons of olive oil

Dried basil (to taste)

Salt and pepper (to taste)

Directions:

1. First, you combine all salad ingredients in a bowl.
2. After which you whisk together all vinaigrette ingredients and pour over salad.
3. Then you mix well.
4. Make sure you refrigerate before serving.

Poached Egg in Avocado

Ingredients:

One avocado

One egg

Directions:

1. First, you fill a bowl with cold water and crack an egg into water.
2. After which you microwave on low for 2 minutes.
3. After that, you drain egg and set aside.
4. Then you pit the avocado and place the egg in the hole.
5. Finally, you salt and pepper to taste.

Avocado Banana Smoothie

Ingredients:

Banana

2 tablespoons of honey

Avocado (chopped)

Sweet yogurt

Directions:

1. First, you place all ingredients in a blender.
2. Then you add ice to taste and blend until smooth.

Black Bean, Mushroom and Avocado Breakfast Scramble

Ingredients:

¼ cup of diced onion

1 small clove garlic (finely minced)

¼ cup of canned black beans, rinsed (or preferably cooked black beans)

A couple turns freshly ground black pepper

A few cilantro leaves (if you so desired)

2 teaspoons of olive oil

1 cup (about 4 ounces) sliced white button mushrooms

2 large eggs

1/8 teaspoon of kosher salt (plus more to taste)

½ small avocado (diced)

Directions:

1. First, you sauté onion and mushrooms in olive oil until softened, about 5 minutes.
2. After which you add garlic and cook for another minute.
3. After that, you crack eggs into small bowl and whisk.
4. At this point, you pour over veggies.
5. Then you add black beans, salt, and pepper.
6. This is when you stir constantly until eggs are cooked.
7. Furthermore, you add salt and pepper to taste.
8. Finally, you scoop on plate and top with diced avocado and cilantro leaves.

Calming Creamy Turmeric Tea

Ingredients

½ teaspoon of turmeric

¼ teaspoon of ginger

1 cup of almond milk

1 teaspoon of cinnamon

1 teaspoon of honey

Directions

1. First, you heat almond milk in the microwave.
2. After which you stir in turmeric, cinnamon, and ginger.
3. Then you drizzle honey on top.
4. Enjoy!

Kale and Blueberry Salad

Ingredients

Ingredient for Salad:

1 cup of fresh blueberries

½ cup of pomegranate seeds

⅓ cup of sliced almonds (toasted)

Salt and black pepper (freshly ground)

3 bunches of kale (stemmed and chopped)

2 medium carrots (peeled and shredded)

⅓ cup of pumpkin seeds (toasted)

1 Tablespoon of chopped fresh mint leaves

½ cup of Soy-Sesame Vinaigrette

Ingredients for Soy-Sesame Vinaigrette:

2 tablespoons of garlic (chopped)

¼ cup of toasted sesame oil

1 cup of rice vinegar

½ cup of soy sauce

2 Tablespoons of water

2 Tablespoons of peeled, chopped fresh ginger

Pinch of red pepper flakes

¼ cup of peanut oil

½ cup of mirin

½ cup of sugar

2 Tablespoons of cornstarch

Directions

Directions to make salad:

1. First, you combine the kale, pomegranate seeds, pumpkin seeds, blueberries, carrots, almonds, and mint in a medium bowl and toss well.
2. After which you drizzle with the vinaigrette and toss again.
3. Then you season to taste with salt and pepper and serve right away.

Direction to make Soy-Sesame Vinaigrette:

1. First, you combine the ginger, sesame oil, garlic, red pepper flakes, and peanut oil in a blender and puree until creamy.
2. After which you pour the mixture into a medium sauté pan and cook, stirring, over low heat until aromatic and golden in color, about 6 minutes.
3. After that, you add the vinegar, soy sauce, mirin, and sugar to the sauté pan.
4. Then you combine the cornstarch and water in a small bowl and then stir the cornstarch slurry into the contents of the pan.
5. At this point, you set the pan over low heat and bring the mixture to a boil to thicken, stirring to dissolve the sugar, about 2 minutes.
6. Finally, you transfer the dressing to a bowl and let cool.
7. Then you cover and refrigerate for up to 1 week.

Fat-Free Refried Bean Recipe

Ingredients (choose organic ingredients when available):

1/3 cup of onion (finely chopped)

½ teaspoon of fresh cilantro or parsley (finely chopped)

1 ½ cups of cooked pinto beans or preferably 1 (about 15 ounces) can organic pinto beans, drained and rinsed

1 ½ tablespoons of fresh lime juice

3 tablespoons of rice vinegar

½ teaspoon of ground cumin

Pinch cayenne pepper

½ cup of coconut water

Directions:

1. First, in a medium saucepan over medium heat, add onion and vinegar and sauté until onions are translucent.
2. After which you stir in cumin, cilantro (or parsley) and pepper and cook for about 30 seconds.
3. After that, you add beans and stir in coconut water.
4. Then you remove from heat and place in a bowl.
5. At this point, you stir in lime juice and with a fork mash some of the beans.
6. This Is when you serve as a spread or make your own quesadillas with whole wheat wraps.
7. Finally, you serve with chopped tomatoes and shredded romaine lettuce.

Baked Cod Fish Recipe

Ingredients:

3 tablespoons of plain nonfat Greek yogurt

1 teaspoon of prepared white horseradish

2 tablespoons of breadcrumbs

Non-stick cooking spray

4 cod fillets (6 ounces each)

1 tablespoon of Dijon mustard

1 teaspoon of fresh dill or ½ teaspoon of dried dill

1 teaspoon of extra virgin olive oil

Directions:

1. Meanwhile, you heat oven to 350 degrees Fahrenheit.
2. After which you coat a large baking dish with non-stick cooking spray.
3. After that, you place fish fillets in dish and turn under thin ends so fillets are an even thickness.
4. Then you mix the mustard, yogurt, horseradish, and dill in a small bowl.
5. At this point, spread evenly over cod and sprinkle with breadcrumbs.
6. This is when you drizzle with the olive oil.
7. Finally, you bake for about 20 minutes or until cooked through.

Yogurt & Chive Dip Recipe

Ingredients:

½ cup of low fat sour cream

1 teaspoon of fresh dill (minced)

sea salt and freshly ground black pepper to taste

1 cup of plain nonfat Greek yogurt

1 tablespoon of fresh lemon juice

1 clove garlic (minced)

2 tablespoons of fresh chives (minced)

Directions:

1. First, in a small mixing bowl, using a whisk, combine the yogurt, dill, garlic, sour cream, lemon juice, and chives until smooth.
2. After which you mix, season with salt and pepper to taste.
3. Then you serve with assorted crudités.
4. Makes about 6 serves.

Healthy Vegetable Focaccia Recipe

Ingredients:

1 pound of whole wheat pizza dough

½ cup of mushrooms (sliced)

¼ teaspoon of coarse sea salt

1-teaspoon of fresh basil (chopped)

2 tablespoons of extra-virgin olive oil

1 cup (about 6 ounces) of organic cherry tomatoes (halved)

1 yellow or orange pepper (cored and diced)

1-teaspoon of fresh Italian parsley (chopped)

Directions:

1. Meanwhile, you heat oven to 400°F.
2. After which you pour oil into a 9-inch-round nonstick cake pan and spread to coat.
3. After that, you place dough into the pan and use your hands to gently stretch the dough.
4. Then you flip dough over so both sides are coated with oil and stretch dough evenly covers the bottom of the pan.
5. At this point, you press tomatoes cut side down into the dough.
6. Furthermore, you top with mushrooms and peppers.
7. After that, you sprinkle with salt, parsley, and basil.
8. After which you bake until the top is brown about 35 to 40 minutes.
9. At this point, cool bread in the pan 5 minutes, then remove and place on a rack.
10. Finally, you serve warm or at room temperature.
11. Make sure you store in an airtight container for up to 1 day.

Beyond Colorado Striped Bass

Ingredients:

½ teaspoon of onion powder

¼ teaspoon of black pepper

Olive oil cooking spray

1 cup of buttermilk (or fat-free milk), preferably organic

½ teaspoon of garlic powder

1- ½ cups of organic corn flakes

1- ½ pounds of hybrid striped bass fillets

Directions:

1. Meanwhile, you heat oven to 450 degrees F.
2. After which you line a baking sheet with foil and coat with cooking spray.
3. After that, combine milk and seasonings in a large bowl.
4. At this point, you place corn flakes in a plastic bag and crush with a rolling pin.
5. Then you place the crumbs on a flat plate.
6. Furthermore, you dip fish fillets into seasoned milk and then roll in crumbs.
7. After that, you place fillets on the baking sheet.
8. This is when you coat the tops of the fillets with a light layer of cooking spray.
9. Then you bake for 12 minutes or until fish flakes easily with a fork.
10. Finally, you serve with your favorite steamed seasonal green vegetable and baked sweet potato.

Easy Irish Soda Bread Rolls (Yeast-Free)

Ingredients:

1-cup of organic all-purpose flour

½ teaspoon of sea salt

2 teaspoons of fresh rosemary (chopped)

1 cup of organic whole-wheat flour

½ teaspoon of baking soda

1 cup of low-fat buttermilk

2 teaspoons of organic sugar

Directions:

1. Meanwhile, you heat oven to 375 degrees Fahrenheit.
2. After which you spray a non-stick baking sheet with cooking spray and set aside.
3. Whisk the dry ingredients in a large bowl.
4. After that, you whisk the wet ingredients in a medium bowl.
5. Then you add the wet ingredients into the dry ingredients and stir until dough forms.
6. Furthermore, on a clean work surface dusted with flour, pat out the dough until 1-inch thick.
7. After which you cut the dough into six 2 ½ -inch rounds.
8. Finally, you place each round on the non-stick baking sheet and bake for about 20 to 25 minutes or until done.
9. Make sure you serve warm.

Strawberry and Chia Pudding

Ingredients

1 (150 g) cup strawberries, thinly sliced

3 tablespoons of chia seeds

1 (about 250 mL) cup of soy beverage, unsweetened, fortified

Directions:

1. First, you mix the chia seeds and soy beverage in a bowl.
2. After which you chill for at least 30 min, or until a pudding consistency is obtained.
3. After that, you mix a few times, to prevent chia seeds from sticking together.
4. Note: if you prefer a smooth consistency, I suggest you blend together the chia seeds and soy beverage using a food processor then chill.
5. In the meantime, thinly slice the strawberries lengthwise; set aside.
6. Finally, you pour the chia seeds pudding into glasses, alternating with the strawberries.
7. Then you serve.

Quinoa and Lentil Salad

Ingredients

2/3 (about 110 g) cup green-brown lentils (dried)

1 (about 180 g) cup quinoa

2 (about 500 mL) cups water

1 (about 200 g) yellow or red sweet peppers, finely diced

1 (about 40 g) shallots, finely chopped

½ (about 70 g) bunch arugula, coarsely chopped

¼ (about 65 mL) cup of extra virgin olive oil

¼ cup lemon juice (freshly squeezed)

1 ½ lemon

2 (10 mL) teaspoons of Dijon mustard

80 g feta cheese (crumbled)

4 (about 12 g) tablespoons of fresh mint, finely chopped

1 (0.1 g) pinch salt [it is optional]

Ground pepper to taste [optional]

Directions:

1. First, you rinse the lentils and cook them in a saucepan of boiling salted water, about 30 min until tender but still somewhat firm.
2. After which you drain, discard the liquid and set aside the lentils.
3. Then you cook the quinoa in the water then let it cool down for 10 minutes.

Directions on how to prepare the vegetables:

1. First, you seed, core and dice the pepper; finely chop the shallot; coarsely chop the arugula.
2. After which you place the vegetables in a large bowl.
3. After that, you add the lentils and quinoa to the bowl.
4. Whisk together the oil, mustard, lemon juice, salt, and pepper in a small bowl.
5. Pour over the salad and gently toss to combine.
6. Then you coarsely crumble the feta cheese and add it on top of the salad.
7. Finally, you sprinkle with the finely chopped mint then serve.

Vegetarian Chili with Tofu

Ingredients

2 cloves garlic (minced)

1 (100 g) carrots, finely diced

½ (70 g) green peppers, finely diced

1 (3 g) teaspoon of ground cumin

1 ¼ (240 g) cup firm regular tofu, finely diced

1 ½ (380 g) cup canned tomatoes (diced)

1/3 (24 g) cup Cheddar cheese, grated

2 (4 g) tablespoons of fresh cilantro [it is optional]

1 (200 g) onions, finely chopped

½ (0.4 g) dried chili peppers, minced

1 (70 g) stalk celery, finely diced

3 (45 mL) tablespoons of canola oil

1 (12 g) tablespoon of brown sugar

1 2/3 (420 mL) cup red beans (canned)

½ (125 mL) cup water approximately

1 (0.1 g) pinch of salt [it is optional]

Ground pepper to taste [it is optional]

Note: before you start I suggest you keep the serving plates in the oven at the lowest setting so they are warm when you serve.

Directions to prepare the vegetables:

1. First, you chop the onion, celery, mince the garlic and chili pepper, finely dice the carrots, and bell pepper.
2. After which you heat the oil in a pan over medium heat.
3. After that, you sauté the onion and garlic about 2 minutes until the onion is translucent, with occasional stirring, paying attention not to let them burn.
4. Then you add the carrots, celery, and bell pepper, then cook for about 4-5 min, with occasional stirring.
5. At this point, you add the minced chili pepper, cumin, and brown sugar, then cook 1 min, with stirring.
6. This is when you finely dice the tofu then add it to the mixture, cook for about 8-10 minute until golden-brown.

7. Furthermore, you drain the beans, rinse them and drain again.
8. After that, you add them to the pan, mix well, add the diced tomatoes and enough water to provide a moist environment.
9. Then you cover and cook over low heat an additional 10 minute until the carrots are tender.
10. Remember, to add salt and pepper to taste.
11. Finally, you sprinkle with freshly chopped cilantro leaves, grated cheddar and serve.

Slow Cooker Shredded Chicken Tex-Mex

Ingredients

½ (100 g) onions, finely chopped

1 clove garlic (minced)

2/3 (about 170 g) cup of canned tomatoes, diced

1 (8 g) tablespoon of ground cumin

1 (0.1 g) pinch cayenne pepper

1 (2 g) tablespoon of dried oregano

1 (4 g) teaspoon of salt

1 (3 g) teaspoon of ground pepper

2 (600 g) chicken breasts, boneless, skinless

1 2/3 cup red beans (canned), rinsed and drained

1 (120 g) cup frozen peas

NOTE: a slow cooker is needed to make this recipe.

Directions:
1. First, you add the first 8 ingredients to the ceramic cooking pot, then mix well.
2. After which you add the chicken and coat it well with the mixture.
3. After that, you cover the slow cooker with the lid and cook on 'low' for about 6-8 h, or until the chicken meat is tender enough to be "pulled" apart easily with a fork.
4. On the other hand, you cook on high for 4-5 hours.
5. Then you take the chicken out of the pot, shred it then put it back into the pot.
6. Finally, you add the beans and peas.
7. At this point, you cover, then cook 10 additional minutes on 'high'.

Avocado, Mango and Grilled Chicken Salad

Ingredients

¼ (35 g) red onions, thinly sliced

1 (300 g) chicken breasts, boneless, skinless

1 (15 mL) tablespoon milk, partly skimmed, 2%

1 (14 g) tablespoon of yogurt, plain, 2%

¼ (1 g) teaspoons of curry powder

1 ½ (23 mL) tablespoons of rice vinegar

2 (30 mL) tablespoons of canola oil

½ (2.5 mL) teaspoon of sesame seed oil

1 (300 g) mangoes, diced

1 (170 g) avocados, diced

1 green onions/scallions (sliced)

1 (0.1 g) pinch salt [it is optional]

Ground pepper to taste [it is optional]

Directions:

1. First, you thinly slice the onion, then soak it in a small bowl filled with water and a few drops of vinegar.
2. After which you set aside while preparing the rest of the salad or leave it overnight in the refrigerator.

(NOTE: this makes the raw onion easier to digest and crispier.)

3. Meanwhile, heat the grill or the broiler.
4. Mix well the yogurt, milk, and curry in a bowl.
5. After that, you brush the chicken breasts with this mixture, then grill or broil 10 cm from the heat.
6. Then you cook for about 10-12 min, turning them once. (NOTE: they are ready when the meat loses its pink color.)
7. At this point, you take out of the oven, add salt and pepper, then slice into strips; set aside.
8. Furthermore, while the chicken is cooking, mix the rice vinegar, pepper, salt, canola and sesame oil in a large bowl.
9. After that, you whisk using a fork until the vinaigrette is well emulsified.
10. After which you drain the onion and add it to the bowl.
11. Then you cut the mangoes in half, without peeling them, slicing near the large oval pit.
12. Make check pattern incisions using a knife (about 1 cm wide) in the flesh without cutting through the skin.

13. This is when you gently press the scored halves to turn them inside out and then cut off the cubes of fruit from the peel.
14. After which you trim the rest of the fruit off the pit.
15. Then you place the mango pieces in the bowl.
16. At this point, you cut the avocados in half and remove the stone, then using a melon-baller, spoon out small balls and add them to the bowl. (NOTE: If a melon-baller is not available, simply dice the avocados).
17. Finally, you add the chicken and sliced green onions, then toss delicately to coat well with the vinaigrette.
18. Must be served right away.

Huevos Rancheros

Ingredients

2 (90 g) corn tortillas

4 eggs size large

2 (30 mL) tablespoons of Fresh Tomatillo Salsa

Ground pepper to taste [it is optional]

 aluminum foil

1 (15 mL) tablespoon of olive oil

2 servings Mexican Rice and Beans

1 (0.1 g) pinch salt [it is optional]

NOTE: Meanwhile, keep the serving plates warm on the stove while you're preparing the dish

Directions:

1. Meanwhile, you heat the oven to 205ºC/400ºF.
2. After which you wrap tortillas in foil, then heat 5 minutes in the oven.
3. After that, you wrap tortillas in clean kitchen towel to keep them warm.
4. On the other hand, heat tortillas over medium heat In a dry hot pan until warmed and lightly toasted.
5. At this point, you heat the oil in a skillet over medium heat.
6. After that, you crack the eggs into the skillet, taking care to keep the yolks intact.
7. Then you cook them sunny-side up or over easy until the whites are firm but the yolks are still runny about 4 minutes.
8. Furthermore, you add salt and pepper to taste.
9. After which you place one tortilla on each warmed plate.
10. This is when you carefully slide two eggs on top of each tortilla.
11. Finally, you add the Mexican Rice and Beans and the Fresh Tomatillo Salsa then serve.

Grilled Eggplant Niçoise Recipe

Ingredients:

1 large eggplant (sliced into thick slabs)

¼ teaspoon of cracked black pepper

½ teaspoon of saffron

1 small fennel bulb (sliced)

¼ cup of sliced pitted Niçoise olives or preferably green olives

4 cloves garlic

Juice of 4 lemons (about ½ cup)

1 tablespoon of dried lavender

4 large slices French bread or sourdough bread (toasted)

2 tomatoes (sliced)

Directions:

1. First, you smash the garlic and rub each slab of eggplant with the garlic.
2. After which you place the eggplant in a shallow bowl and pour the lemon juice over it.
3. After that, you add enough water to submerge the eggplant.
4. Then you allow the eggplant to marinate for at least 1 hour, then drain and place it in a shallow dish.
5. At this point, you add the garlic, pepper, lavender, and saffron and let it sit for about 1 hour.
6. Furthermore, you place the eggplant directly on a grill over medium heat and cook until it is soft on both sides but not charred.
7. Finally, you place a grilled slab of eggplant on a slice of bread and top with a couple slices of fennel and tomatoes and about 1 tablespoon sliced olives.
8. Remember this sandwich is served open faced.

Minted Fruit Kebabs Recipe

Makes 4 kebabs (4 servings)

Ingredients:

4 large strawberries

4 (1-inch-square) honeydew chunks

4 (1-inch-square) watermelon chunks

2 teaspoons of fresh lime juice

4 (10-inch) bamboo skewers

8 red or green grapes

4 (1-inch-square) cantaloupe chunks

4 (½ -inch-thick) slices peeled kiwi

¼ cup of orange juice

2 tablespoons of finely chopped fresh mint leaves

1 teaspoon of pure vanilla extract

Directions:

1. First, you thread 1 grape, 1 honeydew chunk, 1 slice kiwi, 1 strawberry, 1 cantaloupe chunk, 1 watermelon chunk, and 1 more grape onto a skewer.
2. After which you repeat with the remaining fruit and skewers.
3. After that, you place the finished skewers in a shallow container.
4. Whisk together the orange juice, mint, lime juice, and vanilla in a small bowl.
5. Then you pour the marinade over the fruit kebabs, cover, and chill for at least 30 minutes (or better still up to 3 hours) in the refrigerator before serving.

Sweet Potato Burritos Recipe

Serves 4

Ingredients:

1 cup of frozen corn kernels

1 teaspoon of very thinly sliced green onion

1 teaspoon of chili powder

4 (8-inch) whole-wheat tortillas, warmed

2 cups of shredded lettuce

2 cups of peeled and diced sweet potatoes

1 (15-ounce) can low-sodium black beans, drained and rinsed

1 tablespoon of fresh lime juice

Sea salt and freshly ground black pepper

1 cup of prepared salsa

Directions:

1. First, you place the sweet potatoes in a medium saucepan and add water to come an inch up the sides.
2. After which you place over medium-high heat and bring to a boil; cook for 5 minutes, or until the sweet potatoes are tender.
3. After that, you add the corn and cook 1 more minute.
4. Then you drain and transfer to a large bowl.
5. At this point, you add the black beans, lime juice, green onion, and chili powder.
6. Season with salt and pepper to taste.
7. Finally, you divide the filling among the tortillas, top with the salsa and lettuce, roll them up, and serve.

Super Raspberry Protein Brownies Recipe

Makes about 16 brownies

Ingredients:

2 (15-ounce) cans low sodium black beans, drained and rinsed

1 cup of all-fruit raspberry jam

¼ cup of whole-wheat pastry flour

¼ teaspoon of sea salt

¼ teaspoon of safflower oil

1 cup of pitted dates

1 tablespoon of pure vanilla extract

1 cup of unsweetened cocoa powder

Directions:

1. Meanwhile, you heat the oven to 350 F and grease an 8x8-inch baking pan with the oil.
2. After which you combine the black beans, jam, dates, and vanilla in a food processor and process until smooth.
3. After that, you add the flour, cocoa powder, and salt and process again.
4. At this point, you pour into the prepared pan and smooth the top with a spatula.
5. Then you bake for 30 minutes or until the top looks set.
6. Finally, you remove from the oven and cool completely, then cut into 16 squares. (NOTE: The brownies will keep, refrigerated in a covered container, for up to 1 week).

Salad Latine Recipe

As a main dish, it serves 2 or 4 as a side

Ingredients:

3 cloves garlic

4 Roma tomatoes (diced)

¼ cup of pecan halves

½ teaspoon of freshly ground black pepper

½ small white onion

Leaves from 1 bunch chard

1 ½ cups fresh corn kernels

1 cup of seedless black grapes

Pinch of sea salt

Ingredients:

1. First, you mince the onion and garlic, then smash them together a couple times with the back of a knife or with a mortar and pestle.
2. After which you wash the Swiss chard thoroughly, as it tends to be gritty, then slice it into ribbons by tightly bunching the leaves together and slicing them with a sharp, heavy knife.
3. Then you place the chard in a salad bowl, add the remaining ingredients, and toss.

Blueberry Buckwheat Pancakes

Serves 2 to 4

Ingredients:

½ cup of whole-wheat pastry flour

1 teaspoon of aluminum-free baking powder

1 cup of rice milk

Warmed maple syrup (for drizzling)

½ cup of buckwheat flour

2 teaspoons of flaxseed meal

Pinch of sea salt

1 cup of fresh blueberries

1-2 teaspoons safflower oil (to brush the skillet)

Directions:

1. First, you combine the buckwheat flour, baking powder, whole-wheat pastry flour, flaxseed meal, and salt in a medium bowl.
2. After which you whisk briefly to blend.
3. After that, you slowly stir in the rice milk and stir just until the lumps disappear.
4. At this point, you gently fold in the blueberries.
5. Then you heat a cast-iron griddle or skillet over medium heat, then lightly brush with a little of the safflower oil.
6. Furthermore, you add enough batter to form a 4-inch pancake and cook until the edges look dry and bubbly about 2 to 3 minutes.
7. Finally, you gently flip the pancake and cook on the other side until golden, about 2 to 3 minutes.
8. Make sure you serve hot, with warmed maple syrup.

Stuffed Peppers Recipe

As a main dish serves 2 or 4 as a side

Ingredients:

1 cup of cooked black beans

6 green onions (sliced)

2 cloves garlic (minced)

2 tablespoons of apple cider vinegar

¼ teaspoon of sea salt

2 red bell peppers (cut in half, cored, and seeded).

½ cup of cooked brown rice

2 Mexican gray squash or preferably zucchini, diced

2 teaspoons of pepitas (green pumpkin seeds)

1 tablespoon of chopped fresh oregano

Juice of 1 lime

½ teaspoon of freshly ground black pepper

Optional: Salsa

Directions.

1. First, you combine the rice, green onions, pepitas, beans, squash, garlic, oregano, salt, vinegar, lime, and pepper In a large bowl.
2. After which you fill the pepper halves with the squash, rice, and bean mixture.
3. Then you top with salsa, if using, and serve.

Banana Split Oatmeal

Yield: 1 serving

Ingredients:

1/8 teaspoon salt

½ cup of frozen yogurt (non-fat)

1/3 cup of oatmeal, quick-cooking (dry)

¾ cups of water (very hot)

½ banana (sliced)

Directions:

1. First, in a microwave safe cereal bowl, you mix together the oatmeal and salt.
2. After which you stir in water.
3. After that, your microwave on high power for 1 minute; stir.
4. At this point, your microwave on high power for another minute; stir again.
5. Then you microwave an additional 30-60 seconds on high power until the cereal reaches the desired thickness; stir again.
6. Finally, top with banana slices and frozen yogurt.

Healthy Breakfast Frittata

Serves 2

Ingredients:

4 medium cloves garlic (chopped)

1 + 2 Tablespoon of chicken broth

Salt and black pepper (to taste)

½ medium onion (minced)

¼ lb. ground lamb or preferably turkey

3 cups of rinsed and finely chopped kale (stems removed)

5 omega-3 enriched eggs

Directions:

1. First, you mince onion and chop garlic; let them sit for about 5 minutes to enhance their health-promoting benefits.
2. Meanwhile, you heat the broiler on low.
3. After which you heat 1 Tablespoon broth in a 9-10-inch stainless steel skillet.
4. After that, you sauté onion over medium heat, for about 3 minutes, stirring often.
5. Then you add garlic, ground lamb or turkey, and cook for another 3 minutes on medium heat, breaking up clumps.
6. At this point, you add kale and 2 Tablespoons of broth.
7. This is when you reduce heat to low and continue to cook covered for about 5 more minutes.
8. Furthermore, you season with salt and pepper and mix.
9. After that, you beat eggs, season with a pinch of salt and pepper, and pour on top of mixture evenly.
10. After which, you cook on low for another 2 minutes without stirring.
11. Finally, you place skillet under the broiler in middle of oven, about 7 inches from the heat source so it has time to cook without the top burning.
12. Remember, as soon as the eggs are firm, it is done, about 2-3 minutes.

Crustless Spinach Pie

Yield: 2 servings

Ingredients

2 large eggs

½ cup of milk (1%)

½ teaspoon of baking powder

2 cups of spinach (chopped, fresh)

2 tablespoons of butter

½ cup of flour

2 garlic cloves (minced, or ½ teaspoon garlic powder)

4 ounces of mozzarella

Directions:

1. Meanwhile, you heat oven to 350 degrees.
2. After which you melt butter or margarine in an 8-inch baking pan.
3. After that, you beat eggs well.
4. Then you add flour, garlic, milk and baking powder.
5. At this point, you pour into baking pan.
6. Furthermore, stir in cheese and spinach.
7. Finally, bake for 30-35 minutes or until firm and the cheese is slightly golden brown.

Greek Yogurt Parfait
Yield: 4 servings

Ingredients

1 teaspoon vanilla extract

1/4 cup shelled, unsalted dry-roasted chopped pistachios

3 cups plain fat-free Greek-style yogurt (such as Fage)

4 teaspoons honey

28 clementine segments

Directions:

1. First, you combine yogurt and vanilla in a bowl.
2. After which you spoon 1/3 cup yogurt mixture into each of 4 small parfait glasses; top each with ½ teaspoon honey, 5 clementine sections, and ½ tablespoon nuts.
3. After that, you top parfaits with the remaining yogurt mixture (about 1/3 cup each); top each with ½ honey, 2 clementine segments, and ½ tablespoon nuts.
4. Then you serve immediately.

Breakfast Barley with Banana & Sunflower Seeds

Yield: 1 serving

Ingredients

1/3 cup of uncooked quick-cooking pearl barley

1 teaspoon of honey

2/3 cup of water

1 banana (sliced)

1 tablespoon of unsalted salted sunflower seeds

Directions:

1. First, you combine 2/3 cup water and barley in a small microwave-safe bowl.
2. After which you microwave on HIGH 6 minutes.
3. After that, you stir and let stand 2 minutes.
4. Finally, you top with banana slices, sunflower seeds, and honey.

Chinese Chicken Cabbage Salad

Yield: 1 serving

Ingredients:

1 tablespoon of extra virgin olive oil

1 teaspoon of soy sauce

1 medium clove garlic (pressed)

4 oz. of cooked chicken breast (shredded or cut into 1" cubes)

4 cups of Napa cabbage (sliced thin)

1 Tablespoon of rice vinegar

1 tablespoon of minced ginger

2 Tablespoons of chopped cilantro

Directions:

All you do is toss all ingredients together and serve.

Greek Salad

Yield: 1 serving

Ingredients:

2 Tablespoons of chopped mint

2 Tablespoons of chopped olives

1 Tablespoon of extra virgin olive oil

sea salt and pepper (to taste)

4 cups of salad greens

3 Tablespoons of crumbled feta cheese

½ cup of garbanzo beans

1 Tablespoon of red wine vinegar

Directions:

1. First, you combine the salad greens, chopped mint, crumbled feta cheese, olives, garbanzo beans.
2. Then you toss with olive oil and vinegar and add salt and pepper to taste.

Mediterranean Tabouli Salad

Yield: 4 servings

Ingredients:

½ medium onion (minced)

3 cups of minced fresh parsley

3 Tablespoons of extra virgin olive oil

sea salt and pepper (to taste)

1 cup of wheat bulgur (dry), NOTE: makes 2 cups after combining with liquid

2 cloves garlic (pressed or chopped)

1 medium tomato (chopped)

1 Tablespoon of fresh lemon juice or wine vinegar

Directions:

1. First, you place 1 cup wheat bulgur and salt to taste in a bowl.
2. After which you pour 2 cups boiling water or broth over the bulgur, stir once and let sit for about 15-20 minutes until liquid is absorbed.
3. After that, you mince onion and press or chop garlic and let sit for 5 minutes to bring out their hidden health properties.
4. Then you combine all ingredients and mix well.

NOTE: For added flavor, I suggest you add more olive oil and lemon juice.

Marinated Three-Bean Salad

Yield: 4 servings

Ingredients

1 (8 ounces) can cut green beans

1 onion (medium, thinly sliced and separated into two rings)

8 ounces of Italian salad dressing (fat-free)

1 (8.5 ounces) can lima beans

1 (8 ounces) can red kidney beans

½ cup of bell pepper (chopped sweet green)

Directions:

1. First, you drain the canned beans.
2. After which you peel and slice the onion and separate into rings
3. After that, you combine the lima beans, onion rings, green beans, kidney beans, and green bell pepper in a large bowl.
4. Then you pour the Italian dressing over the vegetables and toss lightly.
5. At this point, you cover the bowl and marinate in the refrigerator for at least one hour. (NOTE: the salad can be left in the refrigerator overnight).
6. Finally, you drain before serving.

Poppy Seed Fruit Salad

Yield: 6 servings

Ingredients

3 tablespoons of poppy seed salad dressing

2 cups of cubed pineapple

12 Boston lettuce leaves

3 tablespoons of orange-mango fat-free yogurt (such as Dannon)

2 cups of halved strawberries

1 cup of honeydew melon balls

1 cup of cantaloupe balls

Directions:

1. First, you combine yogurt and salad dressing in a small bowl; stir well with a whisk.
2. After which you combine strawberries, pineapple, and melon balls in a large bowl, tossing gently.
3. After that, you line each of 6 plates with 2 lettuce leaves; spoon 1 cup fruit mixture onto each plate.
4. Then you drizzle each salad with 1 tablespoon dressing.
5. Then you serve immediately.

Immune-Boost Soup

Ingredients:

½ cup of chopped mushrooms (maitake or portabella)

1 can low-sodium white beans (can be substituted for lima beans)

Salt and pepper (to taste)

1 small yellow onion (diced)

1 head escarole, roughly chopped (can substitute with kale or chard)

1 QT organic low-sodium chicken broth/stock

Directions:

1. First, you sauté diced onions and mushrooms in 1 Tablespoon of olive oil.
2. After which you add broth/stock and beans to the veggie mix.
3. After that, you bring to a boil and then add escarole.
4. Finally, you bring to a simmer, then add salt and pepper to taste.

"Just Veggies" Soup

Ingredients:

1 QT of Whole Foods 365 Low-sodium Chicken Broth

1 carrot (diced)

Salt and pepper (to taste)

1 frozen pkg of Whole Foods 365 Vegetable Medley (or better still your favorite frozen veggie mix)

1 small onion (diced)

2 celery stalk (diced)

2 Tablespoons of pecorino cheese

Directions:

1. First, you sweat diced onion, carrot, celery in 1 tablespoon of olive oil.
2. After which you add frozen veggie mix and 1 QT of chicken broth.
3. Then you bring to a boil and let soup warm.
4. Finally, you add salt and pepper to taste.

NOTE: ladle soup into a bowl and top with pecorino cheese for extra flavor!

Pumpkin Soup

Yield: 4 servings

Ingredients

1 onion (small, or 2 teaspoon onion powder)

1 can pumpkin (15 ounces, plain)

Salt and pepper to taste (it is optional)

1 (15 ounces) can white beans, rinsed and drained

1 cup of water

1 (about 14.5 ounces) can chicken or vegetable broth, low-salt

½ teaspoon of thyme or tarragon

Directions:

1. First, you blend white beans, onion and water.
2. After which in a soup pot, mix bean puree with pumpkin, broth, and spices.
3. Then you cover and cook over low heat about 15 to 20 minutes until warmed through.

Spring Vegetable Soup

Yield: 4 servings

Ingredients

¼ red cabbage (medium head, about 2 cups, finely shredded)

½ cup of canned artichoke hearts (drained and chopped)

2 ½ cups of vegetable juice (low-sodium tomato or)

Salt and freshly ground black pepper (to taste)

1 tablespoon of extra-virgin olive oil

2 ripe tomatoes (medium, seeded and chopped)

1 cup of green peas (frozen or fresh)

1 cup of water

2 teaspoons of dried basil

Directions:

1. First, you heat oil in large soup pot over medium heat.
2. After which you sauté tomatoes, cabbage, artichoke hearts and peas for 10 minutes.
3. After that, you add tomato juice and water.
4. Bring to boil and reduce heat.
5. Add basil and simmer for about 10 minutes, or until all vegetables are tender and soup is piping hot.
6. Finally, you serve in individual serving bowls.
7. Make sure you season to taste with salt and pepper.

Pork, Apple & Miso Noodle Soup

Yield: 4 servings, about 2 cups each

Ingredients

12 ounces of lean ground pork

2 cups of reduced-sodium chicken broth

¼ cup of white miso

1 tablespoon of canola oil

2 tart, firm apples (peeled and chopped)

4 cups of water

8 ounces Udon noodles (preferably whole-wheat)

Directions:

1. First, you heat oil in a large saucepan over medium-high heat.
2. After which you add pork and cook, stirring occasionally, for about 2 minutes until no longer pink on the outside.
3. After that, you stir in apples and cook, stirring occasionally, for about 2 minutes more until just beginning to soften.
4. Then you add broth and water; bring to a boil.
5. At this point, you add noodles and cook according to the package directions, stirring occasionally.
6. Furthermore, when the noodles are almost done, carefully scoop out about ½ cup of the cooking liquid from the pan and combine with miso.
7. Finally, you stir the miso mixture into the soup and remove from the heat.
8. Make sure you serve immediately.

Easy Eggplant Stir Fry

Yield: 4 servings

Ingredients

1 zucchini (thinly sliced)

2 onions (sliced)

2 cups of brown rice (cooked)

2 egg plant (peeled and cubed)

1 cup of green bell pepper (cut into strips)

3 tablespoons of Italian salad dressing (low fat)

2 cups of cherry tomatoes

Directions:

1. First, you place eggplant, onions zucchini, green bell pepper, and salad dressing into a skillet.
2. After which you stir lightly to combine and cook over low heat until tender.
3. After that, you stir in cherry tomatoes and cook for about 3-5 minutes.
4. Then you serve over cooked brown rice.

Oriental Sweet and Sour Vegetables
Yield: 6 servings

Ingredients

1 tablespoon of lemon juice

¼ teaspoon of ginger

1 tablespoon of cornstarch (for thickness)

1 pound frozen stir-fry vegetables (bag)

1 tablespoon of honey

1 teaspoon of light soy sauce

1 cup of pineapple or orange juice

2 teaspoons of oil

Directions:

1. First, you combine all ingredients except vegetables in a bowl, mix and set aside.
2. After which you heat 2 teaspoons of oil in a skillet and add frozen vegetables.
3. After that, you cook for 3-4 minutes or until vegetables are crisp-tender.
4. Then you add sweet and sour sauce and cook for another 2 minutes or until mixture comes to a boil.
5. Make sure you serve immediately. (NOTE: this dish is great over pasta or brown rice).

Roasted Cauliflower

Yield: 8 servings

Ingredients

¼ cup plus 2 tablespoons of extra-virgin olive oil

2 tablespoons of freshly grated parmesan

1 (2-pound) head cauliflower, green leaves trimmed

1 teaspoon of kosher salt

2 tablespoons of fresh minced chives

Directions:

1. First, you put oven rack in middle position and preheat oven to 450°F.
2. After which you lightly oil a 9-inch pie plate or square baking dish.
3. After that, you core cauliflower, leaving head intact, then discard core and put cauliflower head in a pan.
4. Then you drizzle 2 tablespoons olive oil over the top of cauliflower and sprinkle with ½ teaspoon salt.
5. Furthermore, you bake until tender, about 1 to 1 1/4 hours.
6. At this point, you transfer to a serving dish.
7. Whisk together ¼ cup olive oil, grated parmesan, minced chives and black pepper in a small bowl.
8. Finally, you place the cauliflower on a platter and drizzle the chive/cheese/olive oil mixture on top.
9. Make sure you serve immediately.

Skillet Meal

Yield: 4 servings

Ingredients

1 (32 ounces) can stewed tomatoes, no salt added

1 (15 ounces) can white beans, rinsed and drained

oregano, basil, or hot pepper (other spices to taste, optional)

one package mustard greens, or collard greens, spinach, or broccoli (10 ounces, frozen)

1 cup of brown rice (cooked)

pepper (to taste)

Directions:

1. First, you steam greens in the stewed tomatoes using a small pan, pot, or electric skillet on medium-high heat.
2. After which you cook greens 10 to 20 minutes until they are as soft as you like them.
3. After that, you stir gently.
4. Then you add the rice, canned beans, and seasonings.
5. Finally, you cook until heated through.

Quick Black Bean Chili

Yield: 2 servings

Ingredients:

2 cloves garlic (minced or pressed)

1 (15-oz) can diced tomatoes

½ cup of cilantro

1 medium onion (chopped)

2 cups or 1 (15 oz.) can (BPA-free) black beans

1 Tablespoon of chili powder

Directions:

1. First, you chop onions and mince or press garlic and let sit for at least 5 minutes to enhance their health promoting properties.
2. After that, you place all ingredients except cilantro in a pot.
3. Cover, and let simmer for about 20 minutes.
4. Then you top with cilantro and serve.

One-Pan Sautee

Ingredients:

1 skinless, boneless chicken breast, cubed into ½ inch pieces (can be substituted for frozen shrimp)

1 cup of frozen brown rice

1 pkg frozen stir-fry veggie mix (no added sauces or seasonings)

¼ cup of low-fat zesty Italian dressing

Directions:

1. First, in a skillet, cook cubed chicken in 1 Tablespoon of olive oil.
2. After which you add stir-fry veggies to skillet and cook for an additional 2-3 minutes.
3. After that, you add frozen rice to skillet and 1 Tablespoon of water (if needed to allow rice to warm).
4. Then you add dressing, bring to a boil and mix ingredients together until veggies are warmed, but still crisp.

"So Easy" Crock Pot Recipe

Ingredients:

1 (about 16-oz.) can of organic, low-sodium chicken broth

2 carrots cut into 1-inch pieces

1 packet of McCormick's Gourmet Seasoning (Chicken and Potatoes or any other flavor you fancy)

1.5 lb. bag frozen skinless, boneless chicken tenders (no breading)

10-15 baby red potatoes

3 stalks of celery cut into 1-inch pieces

1 small onion (sliced)

Directions:

1. First, you spray Crock Pot with olive oil spray.
2. After which you add cut veggies, frozen chicken tenders, potatoes, broth, a packet of seasoning.
3. After that, you mix all together.
4. Then you cook on low for about 6-8 hours.

NOTE: I suggest you use leftovers for lunch the following day or make into a stew.

Snappy Rice Dish

Yield: 2 servings

Ingredients

½ cup of chicken broth, reduced salt (or use water)

½ can kidney beans (about 7 oz.) or chickpeas, pink beans, kidney beans

pepper (to taste)

1 cup of vegetables, frozen or fresh (cut into bite size pieces)

1 cup of brown rice, cooked, or any other rice

Dill weed (fresh-snipped or dry) (to taste)

Directions:

1. First, you steam fry the vegetables in the chicken broth (or water) using a small pan, pot, or electric skillet, on medium high heat.
2. After which you cook the vegetables the way you like them (firm or soft), stirring gently.
3. After that, you add more broth as needed to keep the vegetables moist.
4. Then you add the rice, canned beans, and seasonings.
5. Finally, you steam fry until heated through.

Pan-Grilled Salmon with Pineapple Salsa

Ingredients

2 tablespoons of finely chopped red onion

1 tablespoon of rice vinegar

Cooking spray

½ teaspoon of salt

1 cup of chopped fresh pineapple

2 tablespoons of chopped cilantro

1/8 teaspoon of ground red pepper

4 (6-ounce) salmon fillets (about 1/2-inch thick)

Directions:

1. First, you combine pineapple, red onion, cilantro, rice vinegar and ground red pepper in a bowl; set aside.
2. After which you heat a nonstick grill pan coated with cooking spray over medium-high heat.
3. After that, you sprinkle fish with salt.
4. Then you cook fish for 4 minutes on each side or until it flakes easily when tested with a fork.
5. Finally, you top with salsa.

Stuffed Green Peppers

Yield: 4 servings

Ingredients

1-pound turkey (ground)

½ cup of onion (peeled and chopped)

black pepper (to taste)

4 green peppers (large, washed)

1 cup rice (uncooked)

1 ½ cup of tomato sauce (no added salt)

Directions:

1. First, you cut around the stem of the green peppers.
2. After which you remove the seeds and the pulpy part of the peppers.
3. After that, you wash, and then cook green peppers in boiling water for five minutes; drain well.
4. At this point, you brown turkey in a saucepan.
5. Then you add rice, onion, ½ cup tomato sauce and black pepper.
6. Furthermore, you stuff each pepper with the mixture and place in casserole dish.
7. After which you pour the remaining tomato sauce over the green peppers.
8. Finally, you cover and bake for 30 minutes at 350 degrees.

Brain-Boosting Eggplant Lasagna

SERVINGS: 8

Ingredients:

2 large egg plants (about 2 lb. total), sliced ¼" thick lengthwise

1 medium yellow onion (chopped)

10 oz. of cremini mushrooms, sliced (about 3½ c)

½ c chopped fresh parsley

6 oz. of shredded dairy-free mozzarella-style cheese (I prefer Daiya Mozzarella Style Shreds)

1 pkg (about 14–16 oz.) firm or better still semi-firm tofu, drained

1 Tablespoon of olive oil

2 cloves garlic (minced)

1 jar (about 24 oz.) marinara sauce

1 Tablespoon of freshly grated lemon zest

Directions:

1. First, you place tofu in a fine mesh strainer over a bowl and set aside.
2. After which you heat oven to 375°F.
3. After that, you arrange eggplant on 2 sheet pans lightly coated with cooking spray.
4. Then you coat eggplant with cooking spray and roast until lightly browned, about 12 minutes.
5. At this point, you heat oil in large skillet over medium heat.
6. This is when you add onion and garlic and cook for about 5 to 6 minutes until soft.
7. Add mushrooms and cook for about 8 minutes until tender.
8. Add marinara sauce (NOTE: reserving ½ cup) and bring to simmer.
9. Cook for about 8 minutes until slightly thickened.
10. Furthermore, you place tofu in a medium bowl with parsley, lemon zest, and half of the cheese.
11. After that, you stir until mixture resembles ricotta.
12. After which you spread the remaining ½ cup marinara sauce evenly in 13" × 9" baking pan.
13. Then you layer one-third of the eggplant in pan, then top with one-third of the tofu mixture and one-third of the marinara sauce; repeat twice.
14. Sprinkle with remaining cheese and then bake for about 25 minutes until eggplant is tender.
15. Then you cool for 20 minutes.
16. Finally, you cut into squares and serve.

Slimming Veggie Omelet Squares

SERVINGS: 6

Ingredients:

3 small carrots (halved crosswise then twice lengthwise)

1 Tablespoon of olive oil

2 teaspoons of chopped fresh thyme

8 large eggs

½ cup of whole milk

4 cups of arugula

1 medium sweet potato (peeled and cut into ½"-thick wedges)

1 medium onion (halved and sliced ¼" thick)

2 Tablespoons of roughly chopped parsley

½ cup 2% plain Greek-style yogurt

2 oz. of goat cheese (crumbled)

2 Tablespoons of grated Parmesan

Directions:

1. First, you heat oven to 400°F.
2. After which you place sweet potato, carrots, and onion in 8" × 8" baking pan.
3. After that, you toss with oil and thyme and season with ¼ teaspoon each kosher salt and black pepper.
4. Roast for about 30 minutes until vegetables are tender.
5. Then you toss with parsley and arrange in an even layer in pan.
6. At this point, you whisk eggs, yogurt, and milk in medium bowl.
7. This is when you pour over vegetables and top with goat cheese and Parmesan.
8. Bake for about 20 minutes until puffed and set.
9. Finally, you remove from oven and let rest for about 5 to 10 minutes before cutting into squares and serving with arugula.

DISCOVER HOW TO LIVE A LIFE FREE FROM ALZHEIMER DISEASE.

I will assure you that if you follow this End to Alzheimer's cookbook properly, you WILL prevent and reverse cognitive decline. Recipes are free from processed food that contains refined carbohydrates (like flour and sugar) because they increase inflammation and cause blood sugar fluctuations.

There is NO DIET out there that provides "A HEALTHY YOU" like the End to Alzheimer's cookbook Diet; GIVE IT A TRIAL!